CHAIR YOGA FOR SENIORS OVER 60

Easy Sitting Exercise For Beginners, Intermediate & Advanced Challenged Older Adults To Reclaim Mobility, Balance, Stability, Strength and Independence

CHLOE WILLIAMS

Copyright © [2024] by [Chloe Williams]

INTRODUCTION

Welcome to Yoga For Seniors, a complete guide designed to empower you to your adventure closer to maintaining power, balance, and energy as you gracefully embrace your golden years.

Aging is a herbal part of lifestyles, and it gives a wealth of studies and expertise. However, it also comes with precise challenges, along with diminished stability and improved danger of falls. This book is here to support you in overcoming those obstacles and embracing a satisfying and lively life-style.

As we age, it is not unusual to observe changes in our bodies and day by day abilities. But relaxation assured, those changes now do not avert the pursuit of a colorful and impartial existence. With the right information, willpower, and customized workouts, you could beautify your stability, flexibility, and common bodily well-being.

Yoga For Seniors isn't just every other workout guide; it's a holistic method to senior fitness that encompasses each of the bodily and mental components of growing older gracefully.

Throughout these pages, we can delve into a numerous range of chair physical activities, tailor-made mainly to meet the unique wishes of seniors. Whether you are a pro health fanatic or just starting your journey toward better balance, this book is full of chair sporting activities suitable for all fitness tiers and abilities.

My number one cognizance can be on sporting activities that fortify the middle, enhance posture, decorate coordination, shed stomach fats and project equilibrium, supporting you to regain and maintain your balance. Each workout is carefully illustrated and accompanied through clean, step-by-step instructions, ensuring that you could carry out them appropriately and efficiently in the comfort of your private home or with the steerage of a qualified health teacher.

But stability extends past simply the bodily; it extends into each thing of lifestyles. We will even discover mindful practices, strain-discount techniques, and wholesome life-style selections that promote mental readability, emotional well-being, and an advantageous outlook on life. After all, a balanced mind contributes notably to a balanced body.

Remember, it's by no means too late to put money into your health and well-being. By incorporating these stability sporting activities into your day by day habitual, you will liberate the capability for more independence, improved self belief, and a renewed sense of pleasure in the simple pleasures of existence.

So, embark on this transformative journey with me. Together, permit's include balance, increase our lives with motion and mindfulness, and find out the path to a happier, healthier, and greater balanced you. Your golden years are yours to experience completely – allow them shine!

Table Of Contents

Chapter 1: Introduction To Chair Yoga

In this chapter, we're going to discover the superb advantages of Chair Yoga for seniors over 60 and guide you on a way to get commenced safely. You'll discover how Chair Yoga can enhance flexibility, power, stability, and general proper-being. We'll also offer recommendations on developing a comfortable and supportive practice area.☐

"Chair Yoga for Seniors Over 60" is all about introducing you to the first-rate international of Chair Yoga and its benefits. As we age, it's crucial to maintain our bodily and mental well-being, and Chair Yoga gives a mild yet effective manner to do that.

We'll discover the numerous advantages of Chair Yoga especially designed for seniors like yourself. We'll delve into how it can improve your flexibility, energy, and stability, which can be essential for retaining an energetic and unbiased way of life. Chair Yoga additionally promotes relaxation, reduces strain, reduces weight, belly fat and complements your usual sense of nicely-being.

I'll manual you via the basics of having begun adequately, ensuring that you have a comfortable and supportive exercise area. I'll provide pointers on right posture, breathing techniques, and the way to alter poses to suit your individual needs and talents. Safety is always a top precedence, so we will cowl precautions for precise conditions and offer tips for working towards Chair Yoga without any pressure or soreness.

By the end of this chapter, you'll have a strong expertise of the advantages of Chair Yoga and feel empowered to begin your own exercise. So get geared up to embark on this interesting journey closer to stepped forward fitness and vitality with Chair Yoga for Seniors Over 60! □

This segment units the level to your exciting adventure into the arena of Chair Yoga and its extremely good advantages.

In the creation, you may be delivered to the concept of Chair Yoga and how it's particularly tailored for seniors like yourself. I'll talk about how Chair Yoga can be an outstanding way to enhance your flexibility, energy, stability, and standard proper-being, all at the same time as practicing in the comfort of a chair.

You'll find out about the precise benefits of Chair Yoga, including its accessibility and adaptability for extraordinary health levels and physical skills. We'll additionally discover how Chair Yoga allows you to beautify your mind-frame connection, lessen pressure, and sell relaxation.

The creation will also cowl important safety issues to ensure a snug and fun practice. We'll manual you via right posture, respiratory techniques, and adjustments for poses to fit your man or woman desires.

So get equipped, This book may be your manual to discovering the transformative strength of Chair Yoga for seniors over 60. I cannot wait to allow you to revel in the pleasure and proper-being that Chair Yoga can convey to your lifestyles! □

What Is Chair Yoga?

Chair yoga is a modified form of yoga that is practiced even when seated on a chair or the usage of a chair for guide. It is designed to make yoga reachable to folks who may also have problem with traditional yoga poses or who have restricted mobility. Chair yoga consists of gentle stretches, respiratory sporting events, and mindfulness strategies, offering a secure and powerful way to improve flexibility, energy, stability, and usual nicely-being. It's a superb practice for seniors, people with physical obstacles, or all people searching out a mild and on hand shape exercise.

Chair yoga is likewise a superb cool way to practice yoga even as sitting on a chair or the usage of it for aid. It's best for those who may discover traditional yoga poses though or have limited mobility. You can still stretch, breathe, and get all the advantages of yoga whilst seated. It's terrific for seniors, humans with physical obstacles, or all people who want a mild and handy exercise option.

Benefits of Chair Yoga for Seniors

☐Let's explore the benefits of Chair Yoga for seniors in greater depth. Chair Yoga offers an extensive range of blessings which can greatly decorate the physical, mental, and emotional well-being of older adults.

1. Improved Flexibility: Chair Yoga enables seniors to grow their flexibility by way of lightly stretching and mobilizing the muscle mass and joints. Regular exercise can lead to accelerated variety of motion, making regular movements simpler and extra comfortable.

2. Enhanced Strength and Balance: Chair Yoga consists of gentle strength-constructing exercises that focus on key muscle businesses. This can assist seniors improve their usual energy and balance, decreasing the chance of falls and selling self assurance in each day's exercise.

3. Better Posture and Alignment: By focusing on right alignment and body cognizance, Chair Yoga enables seniors to improve their posture. This can alleviate soreness and strain on the backbone, mainly to improve general frame mechanics.

4. Stress Reduction and Relaxation: Chair Yoga contains respiratory techniques and mindfulness practices that promote relaxation and stress discount. Seniors can experience advanced intellectual readability, reduced anxiety, and an extra sense of calm.

5. Increased Energy and Vitality: Regular exercise of Chair Yoga can enhance strength levels and enhance basic power. The mild movements and conscious respiration strategies assist seniors experience greater invigoration and rejuvenation.

6. Enhanced Mind-Body Connection: Chair Yoga encourages seniors to be gifted within the second and connect to their bodies. This can foster a deeper thoughts-frame connection, mainly to elevated self-awareness and a more sense of ordinary nice-being.

7. Social Connection: Chair Yoga classes provide an opportunity for seniors to connect to others in a supportive and inclusive environment. This social interaction can fight feelings of isolation and sell an experience of community.

8. Improved Circulation: Chair Yoga carries gentle moves and stretches which can decorate blood glide throughout the frame. This can help improve movement and promote healthier cardiovascular features.

9. Reduced Joint Pain: Chair Yoga offers a low-impact way to alleviate joint ache and stiffness. The mild actions and stretches can help lubricate the joints, lessen irritation, and alleviate discomfort.

10. Enhanced Breathing: Chair Yoga emphasizes deep, aware breathing strategies. This can enhance lung potential, growth oxygen intake, and sell relaxation.

11. Better Sleep: Regular exercise of Chair Yoga can help seniors attain higher sleep styles. The combination of bodily motion, rest techniques, and stress reduction can contribute to advanced sleep first-class.

12. Boosted Mood and Mental Well-being: Chair Yoga releases endorphins, the "experience-suitable" hormones, which could increase mood and beautify overall intellectual well-being. It also can offer an experience of accomplishment and empowerment.

13. Improved Digestion: Certain Chair Yoga poses and moves can stimulate the digestive device, helping in digestion and assuaging not unusual digestive problems including bloating and constipation.

14. Increased Mindfulness and Focus: Chair Yoga encourages seniors to be present inside the moment, cultivating mindfulness and improving cognitive features. This can lead to improved awareness, awareness, and intellectual readability.

15. Adaptability for All Abilities: Chair Yoga may be changed to accommodate numerous bodily capabilities and obstacles. It affords a secure and inclusive exercise that may be loved with the aid of seniors of all fitness stages.

Remember, these are only some of the many advantages that Chair Yoga can offer. As you progress via the book, you'll find out even more methods wherein this practice can definitely impact your lifestyles. □

Precautions and Safety Guidelines

□**When it involves training chair yoga for seniors over 60, it is essential to keep some precautions and safety suggestions in thoughts. Here are some key points to keep in mind:**

1. Consult with a healthcare professional: Before starting any new workout program, it's usually an excellent idea to seek advice from a healthcare professional, especially when you have any pre-present scientific situations or issues.

2. Listen in your body: Pay interest for your body's alerts and best do what feels cushty. Avoid pushing yourself too hard or going beyond your limits. Remember, chair yoga is supposed to be mild and reachable.

3. Use a robust chair: Make positive the chair you're using is strong and steady. Avoid chairs with wheels or ones which might be vulnerable to tipping. It's vital to have a stable and supportive base.

4. Modify poses as wanted: Chair yoga offers changes for exceptional talents. If a pose feels too difficult or causes discomfort, feel free to adjust it or pass it altogether. Your safety and luxury are the pinnacle priorities.

5. Warm-up and cool-down: Begin each session with a mild warm-up to prepare your body for motion. Likewise, end with a fab-all the way down to assist your body loosen up and recover. Incorporate gentle stretches and deep respiratory all through these phases.

6. Breathe and loosen up: Focus on your breath in the course of the exercise. Deep, sluggish respiration can help sell rest, lessen pressure, and decorate the thoughts-body connection.

7. Stay hydrated: Remember to drink enough water earlier than, at some point of, and after your chair yoga exercise. Hydration is crucial for standard proper-being.

8. Dress simply: Wear free, breathable apparel that permits for ease of movement. Avoid apparel that restricts your variety of motion or causes discomfort.

9. Create a secure environment: Clear the place around your chair to make sure there aren't any obstacles or dangers that would motivate tripping or falling. Use a non-slip mat or rug to offer balance.

10. Pace yourself: Take breaks as wished and do not overexert yourself. It's perfectly okay to begin with shorter periods and steadily boom the length and depth of your practice over time.

11. Be aware of any ache or discomfort: If you enjoy any pain, pain, or unusual sensations in the course of your exercise, stop and check what is probably causing it. Adjust your posture or modify the pose to relieve any soreness.

12. Stay linked together with your breath: Throughout your exercise, awareness of deep, conscious breathing. This assists you to stay present, calm, and centered.

13. Use props if vital: If you need extra guidance or stability, feel loose to apply props inclusive of cushions, blankets, or blocks. These will let you preserve proper alignment and make the poses more reachable.

14. Stay regular: Regular exercise is prime to reaping the blessings of chair yoga. Aim for consistency to your exercise, although it's only a few minutes every day.

Remember, chair yoga is a wonderful manner to enhance flexibility, electricity, and usual well-being. By following those precautions and safety suggestions, you can ensure an enjoyable exercise.

Chapter 2:
Chair Yoga Basics

☐Let's dive into the basics of chair yoga for seniors over 60.

Chair yoga is a gentle form of yoga that is practiced at the same time as sitting on a chair or the use of a chair for aid.

Here are a few key elements of chair yoga:

1. **Seated Postures:** Chair yoga makes a speciality of a lot of seated postures that assist stretch and improve specific elements of the frame. These postures can target the neck, shoulders, spine, hips, and legs, promoting flexibility and mobility.

2. **Breathing Exercises:** Deep breathing is an imperative part of chair yoga. It allows calm the mind, lessens strain, and increases consciousness. Simple breathing sports can be practiced even as seated, such as deep belly respiratory or trade nose breathing.

3. **Gentle Stretches:** Chair yoga includes gentle stretches that goal to launch anxiety and increase flexibility. These stretches can target regions just like the neck, shoulders, hips, and legs. Remember to move slowly and mindfully, respecting your body's limitations.

4. **Strength-Building Exercises**: Chair yoga includes sporting events that assist construct energy in numerous muscle businesses. These sports can contain lifting mild weights, the usage of resistance bands, or conducting isometric contractions even as seated.

5. **Balance and Coordination**: Chair yoga also specializes in enhancing stability and coordination via precise sporting activities. These physical games might also contain shifting weight, achieving distinct instructions, or practicing easy standing poses with the aid of the chair.

6. **Relaxation and Meditation**: Every chair yoga session commonly ends with a relaxation or meditation exercise. This lets you unwind, launch pressure, and cultivate an experience of internal peace and nicely-being.

□7. **Another crucial factor of chair yoga is training balance and coordination physical games**: These physical games help improve your stability and decorate your capability to transport with grace and manipulate. By that specialize in moving your weight, attaining in exclusive guidelines, and even attempting simple standing poses with the aid of the chair, you may improve your stability and coordination talents.

8. **As you near the give up of a chair yoga consultation, it is critical to comprise relaxation and meditation:** These practices allow you to unwind, allow movement of stress, and cultivate a deep experience of inner peace and nice-being. You can have interaction in guided relaxation strategies or explore exclusive meditation patterns that resonate with you.

9. **Chair yoga is a customizable practice that may be tailored to suit your precise desires and competencies:** It's all approximately finding comfort and support while nonetheless reaping the blessings of yoga. Always listen to your body, make changes as necessary, and honor your consolation stage. Remember, there's no person-length-suits-all technique to chair yoga.

10. **Chair yoga is obtainable to humans of every age and health degrees:** Whether you are an amateur or were practicing yoga for years, chair yoga offers a gentle yet effective manner to improve your bodily and intellectual well-being. It's an exercise that meets you in which you're and facilitates your development at your own tempo.

11. **Chair yoga isn't always just about the physical blessings;** It additionally promotes mindfulness and a general feel of nicely-being. By connecting with your breath, being a gift within the moment, and cultivating an experience of gratitude, chair yoga permits you to locate balance, lessen pressure, and beautify your universal satisfaction of lifestyles.

12. **Remember, the splendor of chair yoga is that you may practice it whenever, everywhere:** Whether you're at home, inside the workplace, or even at the same time as touring, all you need is a chair and a willingness to discover the practice. So, why not try to enjoy the tremendous advantages of chair yoga for yourself?

Remember, chair yoga is a customizable exercise that may be tailor-made for your character desires and skills. It's constantly critical to listen to your frame, modify poses as wanted, and paintings within your comfort area.

Breathing Techniques for Relaxation and Mindfulness

☐Breathing sporting events are a effective device to help calm the thoughts, lessen strain, and sell a sense of rest. Here are a few techniques you may attempt:

1. **Deep Belly Breathing:** Find a snug seated function, close your eyes, and region one hand for your belly. Take a sluggish, deep breath in via your nostril, permitting your belly to rise as you fill your lungs with air. Then, exhale slowly through your mouth, feeling your belly fall. Repeat this deep stomach breathing for numerous minutes, that specialize in the feeling of your breath.

2. **Four-7-8 Breathing:** This method facilitates adjusting your breath and promotes an experience of calm. Start by exhaling absolutely through your mouth. Then, inhale quietly via your nose to an intellectual matter of four. Hold your breath for a matter of 7. Finally, exhale completely through your mouth to a depend of 8. Repeat this cycle for some rounds, permitting every breath to be gradual and managed.

3. **Box Breathing:** Visualize a container with four equal sides. Inhale slowly thru your nose as you trace the first aspect of the container, counting to four. Hold your breath as you hint at the second one side, counting to four. Exhale slowly through your nose or mouth as you hint at the 1/3 side, counting to four. Finally, preserve your breath once more as you trace the fourth facet, counting to 4. Repeat this box respiration pattern for a few minutes, focusing on the rhythm of your breath.

4. **Alternate Nostril Breathing:** This method allows stability of the electricity on your body and calms the mind. Start by means of sitting readily and the use of your proper hand. Close your proper nostril along with your proper thumb and inhale deeply via your left nose. Then, near your left nose with your ring finger and exhale through your proper nostril. Inhale through your proper nose, then close it and exhale via your left nostril. Continue this alternate nose respiration for a couple of minutes, keeping a consistent and relaxed breath.

Remember, these breathing techniques can be practiced anywhere and at any time while you want a second of relaxation and mindfulness. Feel unfastened to discover and locate the method that resonates with you the most.

Gentle Warm-up Exercises

Warm-up sports are critical to put together your frame for bodily activity and assist prevent accidents. Here are a few gentle heat-up physical activities you may try:

1. **Neck Rolls:** Stand or sit up and slowly roll your head in a round motion, starting with small circles and regularly growing the size. Repeat in the opposite course.

2. **Shoulder Rolls:** Stand along with your ft shoulder-width aside and relax your palms by your aspects. Roll your shoulders forward in a round motion, then roll them backward. Repeat several times.

3. **Arm Circles:** Extend your hands out to the perimeters at shoulder peak. Make small circles with your hands, regularly increasing the size. After a few circles, reverse the course.

4. **Side Bends:** Stand with your toes hip-width aside and locate your arms in your hips. Gently lean to at least one aspect, stretching the alternative side of your body. Hold for a few seconds, then return to the starting function. Repeat on the opposite facet.

5. **Leg Swings:** Stand next to a wall or preserve onto a robust object for assistance. Swing one leg ahead and backward, maintaining it directly. Repeat for 10-15 swings, then transfer to the other leg.

Remember to pay attention in your frame and pass at your personal pace. These mild heat-up exercise activities will assist lighten up your muscle mass and get your blood flowing earlier than any physical hobby.

Seated Stretches for Flexibility

☐Seated stretches are a exquisite way to enhance flexibility, even if you opt to workout even when sitting. Here are some seated stretches you can try:

1. **Seated Forward Bend:** Sit on the threshold of a chair together with your ft flat on the ground. Slowly bend forward from your hips, accomplishing your fingers in the direction of your ft or the floor. Hold the stretch for 15-30 seconds, then slowly sit back up.

2. **Seated Spinal Twist:** Sit up instantly in your chair and pass one leg over the alternative. Place your opposite hand on the outside of your bent knee and gently twist your torso towards that side. Hold the stretch for 15-30 seconds, then repeat on the other side.

3. **Seated Side Stretch:** Sit up straight and reach one arm overhead, leaning toward the other facet. Feel the stretch alongside the facet of your body. Hold for 15-30 seconds, then switch aspects.

4. **Seated Neck Stretch:** Sit up directly and lightly tilt your head to one side, bringing your ear towards your shoulder. Hold for 15-30 seconds, then repeat on the alternative aspect. You can also strive lightly rotating your head to and fro to stretch the neck muscular tissues.

Remember to respire deeply and by no means push yourself too far in any stretch. It's essential to listen to your frame and stop if you feel any ache. These seated stretches can assist enhance flexibility and relieve tension.

Chapter 3:
Chair Yoga Poses

Seated Mountain Pose:

☐To do the Seated Mountain Pose, start through sitting up immediately to your chair with your feet flat at the ground. Place your hands to your thighs or rest them gently in your knees. Close your eyes if you're comfortable doing so.

Take a deep breath in, lengthening your spine, and believe yourself developing tall like a mountain. As you exhale, relax your shoulders and launch any tension in your body.

Keep your posture tall and comfortable as you continue to breathe deeply. This seated variant of the Mountain Pose facilitates grounding and stability.

Seated Forward Fold

To do the Seated Forward Fold, begin with the aid of sitting on the brink of your chair together with your feet flat on the ground. Take a deep breath in, and as you exhale, slowly hinge forward from your hips. Reach your fingers in the direction of your feet or the floor, allowing your head and chest to loosen up ahead. Remember to maintain your returned instantly and avoid rounding your shoulders. Hold the stretch for some breaths, feeling the mild stretch on your hamstrings and lower lower back. If you sense any discomfort, simplest cross as some distance as feels snug for you. Slowly sit again up as you inhale. Seated Forward Fold is a incredible stretch for liberating tension in the lower back and hamstrings.

Seated Twist

☐To do the Seated Twist, start by using sitting up straight for your chair together with your toes flat on the floor. Place one hand on the outdoor of your contrary knee. As you inhale, extend your backbone and take a seat tall. On your exhale, gently twist your torso in the direction of the facet of the hand for your knee, using your hand to help deepen the twist. Keep your gaze over your shoulder if it feels comfortable for your neck. Hold the twist for some breaths, feeling the stretch to your lower back and torso. Inhale to launch the twist and repeat on the opposite side. Seated twists are excellent for improving spinal mobility and releasing tension to your back.

Seated Cat-Cow Stretch

☐To do the Seated Cat-Cow Stretch, start by means of sitting up instantly in your chair with your ft flat on the floor. Place your hands for your thighs or knees. As you inhale, arch your again and lift your chest, allowing your stomach to drop forward. This is the Cow pose. Then, as you exhale, spherical your spine, tuck your chin for your chest, and draw your belly button in in the direction of your spine. This is the Cat pose. Continue flowing between those two poses, breathing in to Cow and exhaling to Cat. Move along with your breath, locating a rhythm that feels appropriate for you.

The Seated Cat-Cow Stretch enables you to mobilize your spine and promote flexibility.

Chapter 4:

Chair Yoga Routine

Morning Energizer Routine

☐Here's a morning energizer recurring that will help you start your day without work with a boost of electricity:

1. Stretch and Yawn: Start by stretching your hands overhead and taking a massive yawn to wake up your frame and thoughts.

2. Deep Breathing: Sit up immediately, close your eyes, and take some deep breaths in thru your nostril and out thru your mouth. Feel the power filling your lungs and invigorating your body.

3. Shoulder Rolls: Roll your shoulders forward and backward numerous times to launch any tension on your top frame and enhance stream.

4. Jumping Jacks: Stand up and do some sets of jumping jacks to get your coronary heart free up and growth blood drift at some point of your frame.

5. High Knees: Stand in vicinity and raise your knees up toward your chest, alternating legs. This exercise facilitates to warm up your leg muscle groups and gets your blood flowing.

6. Sun Salutations: Flow through a few rounds of solar salutations, a sequence of poses that extend and strengthen your whole frame. Modify the poses as hard to accommodate your strength degree and mobility.

7. Dance Break: Put in your favored upbeat music and feature a mini dance birthday celebration to get your body shifting and improve your temper.

8. Hydration: Don't neglect to drink a glass of water to rehydrate your frame after a night time of sleep.

Remember to concentrate on your body and alter the depth of the exercises based on your comfort level. Have a first-rate energizing morning.

Afternoon Stretch and Relax Routine

☐If you're searching out for an afternoon stretch and relax habitual, here's easy ones you can try:

1. Neck Stretches: Gently tilt your head to one aspect, bringing your ear in the direction of your shoulder. Hold for a few seconds, then transfer sides. Repeat a few instances to launch anxiety in your neck.

2. Shoulder and Upper Back Stretch: Interlace your arms in the back of your back and lightly straighten your palms whilst lifting your chest. Feel the stretch for your shoulders and top again. Hold for a few breaths.

3. Spinal Twist: Sit up immediately for your chair and vicinity your proper hand at the outside of your left thigh. Inhale, lengthen your backbone, and exhale as you twist to the left, looking over your left shoulder. Hold for some breaths, then switch facets.

4. Seated Forward Fold: Sit closer to the threshold of your chair, feet flat on the floor. Inhale, prolong your spine, and exhale as

you hinge ahead from your hips, reaching your palms in the direction of your feet or the floor. Feel the stretch for your hamstrings and lower again. Hold for some breaths.

5. Deep Breathing: Close your eyes, take gradual, deep breaths, and awareness of enjoying your body and thoughts. Inhale through your nose, filling your belly with air, and exhale through your mouth, freeing any anxiety.

6. Mindful Break: Take a couple of minutes to practice mindfulness or meditation. Focus on the existing second, letting go of any issues or distractions. Allow yourself to fully relax and recharge.

Remember to concentrate for your body and alter any stretches or physical games to suit your consolation stage. Enjoy your afternoon stretch and loosen up routine.

Bedtime Wind-Down Routine

☐If you are seeking out a bedtime wind-down ordinary, here are some thoughts that will help you loosen up and put together for an excellent night time's sleep:

1. Disconnect from Screens: About an hour earlier than the mattress, place away electronic devices like telephones, capsules, and laptops. The blue mild emitted via displays can interfere together with your sleep quality.

2. Dim the Lights: Create a relaxed and comfortable ecosystem by dimming the lights in your bedroom. This can assist signal to your frame that it is time to wind down and put together for sleep.

3. Gentle Stretching: Engage in some mild stretching or light yoga poses to release any tension in your body. Focus on gradual, planned actions and deep respiration to sell relaxation.

4. Warm Bath or Shower: Take a warm tub or bathe to assist relax your muscular tissues and soothe your mind. You can add

some calming important oils like lavender to enhance the rest impact.

5. Mindfulness or Meditation: Practice mindfulness or meditation strategies to quiet your mind and promote relaxation. Focus on your breath or use guided meditation apps to help you unwind.

6. Reading or Journaling: Engage in a calming activity like reading a book or writing in a magazine. Choose something mild and exciting to help shift your consciousness far from daily stressors.

7. Herbal Tea: Sip on a cup of natural tea like chamomile or lavender. These teas have calming properties that permit you to relax earlier than bed.

8. Create a Bedtime Routine: Establish a consistent bedtime recurring that consists of these wind-down sports. By following the equal routine every night, your frame will start to apprehend the cues and prepare for sleep.

Remember, it is crucial to concentrate on your frame and locate what works great for you. Sweet dreams.

Chapter 5:
Modifying Chair Yoga for Individual Needs

☐Chair yoga can be without problems modified to deal with person desires and talents. Here are some methods to adjust chair yoga poses:

1. **Use Props:** Props like blankets, blocks, or straps can provide aid and make poses more on hand. For instance, the use of a blanket beneath the ft can help with balance in seated poses.

2. **Adjust Seat Height**: If wanted, you can alter the peak of the chair through including cushions or adjusting the seat height to make it extra comfortable for positive poses.

3. **Focus on Range of Motion**: If a person has a confined range of motion, they are able to modify poses by way of decreasing the variety or the usage of smaller moves. The key's to transport inside a snug range without inflicting ache or soreness.

4. **Offer Chair Variations**: Some poses may be accomplished both on and rancid the chair. For example, if a status pose is

challenging, it is able to be changed to a seated version on the chair.

5. **Provide Options for Balance**: If balance is a challenge, inspire using the chair for assistance at some point of status poses. The chair may be used for balance and to save you falls.

Remember, it is important to concentrate on your frame and regulate poses primarily based on your character wishes.

Adapting Poses for Limited Mobility

☐When it comes to adapting poses for constrained mobility, there are numerous changes you can make to ensure a secure and fun chair yoga practice. Here are some suggestions:

1. **Seated Variations**: Many conventional yoga poses may be tailored to a seated role. For instance, in preference to standing ahead fold, you could do a seated ahead fold by way of gently hinging ahead from the hips at the same time as sitting in a chair.

2. **Gentle Stretches:** Focus on gentle stretches that concentrate on unique areas of the frame. For instance, you can do seated neck stretches, shoulder rolls, or wrist and ankle rotations to promote mobility and flexibility.

3. **Use Supportive Props**: Utilize props like blankets, blocks, or cushions to provide extra aid and comfort in the course of poses.

For example, putting a cushion under the knees can assist alleviate strain all through seated poses.

4. **Modify Range of Motion**: Adjust the variety of motion in poses to accommodate constrained mobility. You can lessen the depth of a stretch or movement to a comfortable level that does not cause any soreness or ache.

5. **Incorporate Chair Exercises**: Integrate chair exercises that especially goal electricity and mobility. This can consist of seated leg lifts, seated marches, or seated arm physical activities using resistance bands.

Remember, it is critical to listen to your body and best do what feels comfortable for you. If you have any unique worries or obstacles, it is always an amazing concept to seek advice from a healthcare professional or an authorized yoga instructor who can offer customized steerage.

I wish these suggestions help you adapt poses for restricted mobility during your chair yoga exercise.

Chair Yoga for Chronic Pain Management

☐Chair yoga can be a top notch exercise for dealing with chronic pain. It gives mild moves and modifications that can help alleviate discomfort and promote common properly-being. Here's how chair yoga can be useful for continual ache management:

1. **Gentle Movements**: Chair yoga focuses on gentle actions and stretches that may be modified to suit person desires. These movements assist boom flow, reduce stiffness, and improve joint mobility, which may be particularly beneficial for dealing with persistent ache.

2. **Mind-Body Connection**: Chair yoga carries mindfulness and breath awareness, which could help shift attention far from ache and sell rest. By cultivating a mind-body connection, you could learn how to better manage and deal with chronic aches.

3. **Stretching and Strengthening**: Chair yoga includes a whole lot of seated stretches and energy-building physical games that focus on different regions of the body. Stretching facilitates

relieve anxiety and enhance flexibility, even as strengthening physical activities can help guide and stabilize the frame, decreasing ache and soreness.

4. **Breathing Techniques**: Deep, conscious breathing techniques are a crucial part of chair yoga. These strategies can assist calm the fearful device, reduce strain, and promote relaxation, which may be useful for managing chronic pain.

5. **Adaptability**: Chair yoga may be without problems tailored to deal with various degrees of mobility and ache. It permits modifications and using props to make the exercise greater handy and cushty for people with continual ache.

Remember, it's usually critical to listen to your frame and work inside your comfort level. If you have any precise worries or questions on practicing chair yoga for continual pain, it is a great concept to seek advice from a healthcare professional or a licensed yoga teacher who can offer personalized steering.

I desire this fact to allow you to understand how chair yoga can be a precious tool for coping with continual pain.

Chair Yoga for Seniors with Specific Health Conditions

☐Chair yoga is a awesome option for seniors with unique health conditions. It offers a mild and accessible manner to stay energetic and promote standard well-being.

Here are some examples of ways chair yoga can gain seniors with precise fitness conditions:

1. **Arthritis**: Chair yoga can assist seniors with arthritis by focusing on gentle actions that promote joint mobility, lessen stiffness, and alleviate ache. It also consists of stretching sporting activities which could enhance flexibility and reduce soreness.

2. **Osteoporosis**: Chair yoga can be tailored to accommodate seniors with osteoporosis, specializing in gentle weight-bearing physical activities that assist keep bone density and improve balance. It emphasizes right alignment and includes moves that reinforce the center and decrease frame.

3. **Cardiovascular Health**: Chair yoga may be useful for seniors with cardiovascular conditions by incorporating mild movements that promote circulation and growth heart rate in a safe and managed way. It additionally consists of respiratory

physical games that help lessen pressure and improve normal cardiovascular health.

4. **Diabetes**: Chair yoga can help seniors with diabetes by incorporating mild stretches and actions that promote blood stream and enhance insulin sensitivity. It additionally emphasizes rest strategies which could assist control stress ranges, that is vital for diabetes control.

5. **Chronic Pain**: Chair yoga is a superb alternative for seniors managing persistent ache. It includes gentle movements, stretches, and respiratory physical games that assist alleviate pain, boom flexibility, and sell rest.

Remember, it's critical to seek advice from a healthcare expert before starting any exercising application, mainly if you have particular health situations. They can offer personalized steering and ensure that chair yoga is secure and suitable for your individual needs.

Chapter 6:

Chair Yoga for Daily Living

☐Chair yoga isn't always just for unique fitness conditions, however it is also remarkable for day by day residing. It offers a convenient and available manner to incorporate movement, mindfulness, and relaxation into your normal ordinary. Here's how chair yoga can enhance your daily existence:

1. **Promotes Physical Well-being**: Chair yoga consists of numerous seated postures, gentle stretches, and strength-building physical games that assist enhance flexibility, balance, and overall physical health. It can help alleviate stiffness and discomfort, boom energy degrees, and beautify your range of movement.

2. **Boosts Mental Clarity:** Chair yoga includes breathing exercises and mindfulness techniques that can assist calm the thoughts, reduce stress, and increase intellectual readability. It provides a possibility to cognizance of the present moment, launch anxiety, and enhance your standard sense of nicely-being.

3. **Improves Posture**: Many of us spend a sizable quantity of time sitting, which can result in bad posture and associated problems. Chair yoga consists of sporting activities that promote right alignment and reinforce the muscle mass that assist proper posture. By practicing frequently, you can improve your posture and reduce the risk of soreness or injury.

4. **Increases Energy and Vitality:** Chair yoga contains gentle movements and stretches that stimulate blood flow and power glide at some stage in the frame. By incorporating chair yoga into your daily habit, you could experience improved vitality, progressed mood, and a more feel of typical well-being.

5. **Enhances Relaxation and Stress Relief**: Chair yoga includes rest and meditation techniques that will let you unwind, lessen pressure, and sell an experience of calm. It gives a possibility to disconnect from the busyness of day by day lifestyles and create a space for self-care and relaxation.

Remember, chair yoga can be tailor-made on your person's desires and skills. It's usually a very good idea to pay attention to your body, adjust poses as needed, and work within your consolation area. If you are new to chair yoga, keep in mind finding a qualified instructor or the usage of online resources to guide you through the practice.

Chair Yoga at the Office

☐Chair yoga on the workplace is a terrific manner to comprise movement and relaxation into your workday. Here's how it can advantage you:

1. **Relieve Stress**: Office work may be annoying and demanding. Chair yoga gives a chance to take a ruin, stretch your body, and clean your thoughts. It enables anxiety to your muscle tissues, lessens stress stages, and promotes a feel of calm and cognizance.

2. **Boost Energy and Productivity**: Sitting for long durations could make you feel sluggish and tired. Chair yoga provides mild actions and stretches that increase blood flow, oxygenate your body, and boost strength tiers. By incorporating it into your office recurring, you'll experience greater alert, focused, and effective.

3. **Improve Posture and Prevent Discomfort**: Sitting at a desk for hours can result in negative posture and pain, specially inside the neck, shoulders, and lower back. Chair yoga consists of sports that sell proper alignment, enhance center muscle groups, and improve posture. Regular practice can help alleviate discomfort and decrease the threat of musculoskeletal problems.

4. **Enhance Mental Clarity**: Chair yoga contains breathing techniques and mindfulness sports that assist calm the mind, enhance awareness, and enhance mental clarity. Taking short breaks to practice chair yoga can refresh your mind, boom creativity, and enhance average cognitive characteristics.

5. **Create a Positive Work Environment**: Practicing chair yoga at the workplace can inspire your colleagues to enroll in or take breaks for his or her personal nicely-being. It fosters a supportive and wholesome painting environment, encouraging self-care and selling a tremendous mind-set amongst coworkers.

Remember, you do not need quite a lot of space or a unique system to do chair yoga in the office. Just find a quiet region in which you could conveniently take a seat in your chair and observe some simple poses and stretches. There are masses of online assets and movies available to guide you via office-friendly chair yoga workouts.

Give it an attempt in the course of your work breaks.

Chair Yoga for Travel

☐Chair yoga is a exquisite alternative for staying energetic and relaxed even as traveling. Here's why it's ideal in your travel adventures:

1. **Portable and Convenient**: Since chair yoga can be achieved whilst sitting, it is especially convenient for touring. Whether you are on a plane, teaching, or waiting on the airport, you may effortlessly exercise chair yoga in your seat. No need for a yoga mat or a variety of areas!

2. **Relieve Travel Tension**: Traveling can every now and then be demanding and take a toll on your frame. Chair yoga gives gentle stretches and actions that help launch anxiety in your muscle tissues and promote relaxation. It's an incredible manner to unwind and ease any tour-related pressure.

3. **Improve Circulation**: Sitting for long intervals all through the journey can result in negative circulation. Chair yoga includes physical games that stimulate blood flow and assist prevent stiffness and pain. By practicing chair yoga, you can maintain your frame active and sell better circulation.

4. **Boost Energy**: Traveling may be tiring, especially in case you're coping with jet lag or long journeys. Chair yoga consists of energizing poses and respiration sporting events that could help revitalize your frame and thoughts. It's a natural manner to boost your power levels and stay refreshed all through your travels.

5. **Maintain Flexibility**: Sitting for extended periods can motivate your muscle tissues to tighten up. Chair yoga focuses on mild stretches that assist keep flexibility, even whilst on the go. By incorporating chair yoga into your ordinary journey, you can hold your frame limber and prevent any stiffness.

Remember, you could locate lots of chair yoga resources online that cater in particular to travelers. These routines are designed to be simple, powerful, and suitable for various travel situations. So, whether or not you're on a plane, in a lodge room, or waiting at a bus station, you can revel in the benefits of chair yoga anyplace your travels take you!

Safe and enjoyable travels, my buddy!

Chair Yoga for Improved Posture

☐Chair yoga is an super practice for improving posture. Here's how it may help:

1. **Increased Awareness**: Chair yoga encourages you to emerge as extra aware of your frame and posture. By working towards diverse seated poses, you expand a heightened feel of alignment and learn to recognize whilst your posture needs adjustment.

2. **Core Strengthening**: Many chair yoga poses engage the core muscle mass, including the abdominals and lower back muscular tissues. Strengthening those muscular tissues gives vital help for retaining right posture. As you beef up your core, you'll find it simpler to sit or stand tall with right alignment.

3. **Spinal Alignment**: Chair yoga poses regularly contain mild twists and stretches that assist release tension and promote spinal alignment. By regularly working towards those poses, you may alleviate any imbalances or pain for your spine, leading to stepped forward posture over the years.

4. **Shoulder and Chest Opening**: Sitting for extended durations can cause the shoulders to spherical forward and the chest to

grow to be tight. Chair yoga includes physical games that open up the chest and stretch the shoulders, counteracting the outcomes of slouching and selling an extra open and upright posture.

5. **Mind-Body Connection**: Chair yoga emphasizes the thoughts-frame connection, allowing you to tune into your frame's signals and make modifications in your posture in the course of the day. With multiplied cognizance, you could catch yourself slouching and consciously correct your posture to maintain an extra aligned and upright position.

Remember, consistency is key when it comes to improving posture with chair yoga. Regular exercise will help give a boost to the muscular tissues needed for correct posture and enhance healthful alignment behavior. So, snatch a chair and begin incorporating chair yoga into your every day recurring for a more confident and aligned posture!

Keep up the tremendous paintings!

Chapter 7:

Chair Yoga for Mind-Body Connection

☐Chair yoga is notable for nurturing the mind-body connection. Here's why:

1. **Present Moment Awareness**: Chair yoga encourages you to be absolutely present in the second. As you pass via the mild poses and cognizance on your breath, you become greater attuned to the sensations on your frame. This heightened awareness enables you to connect to your frame and the present moment, fostering a deeper thoughts-body connection.

2. **Breath Awareness**: One of the key components of chair yoga is aware respiration. By paying attention to your breath and engaging in unique respiratory sporting activities, you increase a more potent connection among your breath and your frame. This connection can help calm the mind, reduce strain, and sell ordinary nicely-being.

3. **Mindful Movement**: Chair yoga includes gradual and planned movements, permitting you to engage with every posture mindfully. As you pass through the poses, you can pay attention to the sensations, the alignment of your body, and the breath.

This mindful motion cultivates a deeper connection among your thoughts and body, enhancing your common yoga enjoyment.

4. **Stress Reduction**: Chair yoga offers a gentle and reachable manner to launch pressure and tension. By training relaxation strategies, consisting of guided imagery and meditation, you may calm the thoughts and relax the body. This relaxation reaction facilitates to lessen stress stages and promotes an extra experience of concord among your thoughts and body.

5. **Emotional Well-being**: Engaging in chair yoga can have a fantastic effect on your emotional well-being. The mind-body connection fostered via the exercise can help you come to be more aware about your emotions and offer an area for self-mirrored image. By acknowledging and honoring your feelings for the duration of chair yoga, you could cultivate a greater sense of emotional stability and well-being.

So, through incorporating chair yoga into your habitual, you may reinforce the mind-body connection, decorate your attention, reduce pressure, and promote emotional nice-being. It's a lovely exercise that nourishes each frame and your mind. Give it an attempt to enjoy the excellent advantages!

Keep exploring the terrific world of chair yoga!

Exploring Mindfulness in Chair Yoga

☐Exploring mindfulness in chair yoga is a great way to deepen your exercise. Here's how it could advantage you:

1. **Cultivating Present-Moment Awareness**: Mindfulness is all about being absolutely gifted inside the second. In chair yoga, you could bring mindfulness to every movement, breath, and sensation. By focusing your attention on the present moment, you enhance your thoughts-body connection and deepen your standard yoga experience.

2. **Tuning into Sensations:** Mindfulness invites you to music into the sensations to your frame as you practice chair yoga. Whether it's the stretch on your muscular tissues, the sensation of your breath, or the mild actions, taking note of those sensations facilitates you stay grounded and linked to the present moment.

3. **Observing Thoughts and Emotions**: Mindfulness encourages you to observe your mind and emotions without judgment. As you interact in chair yoga, you could become aware of any mind or emotions that get up during the exercise. By gazing at them without attachment or judgment, you may domesticate an experience of inner calm and acceptance.

4. **Deepening Breath Awareness:** Mindfulness and breath consciousness move hand in hand. In chair yoga, you may convey mindfulness on your breath by means of focusing on its rhythm, depth, and quality. By directing your attention to the breath, you can calm the mind, reduce pressure, and beautify your typical experience of being nicely-being.

5. **Engaging in Mindful Movement**: Chair yoga offers a completely unique possibility to practice aware motion. As you drift via the poses, you could bring your complete interest to the sensations, alignment, and transitions. This aware motion allows you to fully enjoy the advantages of chair yoga and connect more deeply with your frame.

By exploring mindfulness in chair yoga, you may enhance your practice, cultivate a more sense of presence, and enjoy the various blessings of mindfulness to your everyday life. So, include the energy of mindfulness as you interact in chair yoga and enjoy the beautiful journey of self-discovery and internal peace.

Keep exploring and embracing mindfulness to your chair yoga exercise!

Chair Yoga and Emotional Well-being

□Chair yoga may have a profound impact to your emotional properly-being. Here's how it could assist:

1. **Stress Reduction**: Chair yoga carries mild actions, breathing sports, and relaxation strategies that could help lessen stress levels. By focusing on the prevailing moment and attraction in mindful movement, you could release tension, calm your mind, and sell a feeling of internal peace.

2. **Mood Enhancement**: Engaging in chair yoga can launch endorphins, which can be natural temper boosters. The mixture of mild stretches, breathing sporting activities, and rest strategies can help uplift your mood, increase emotions of positivity, and decrease symptoms of hysteria and depression.

3. **Mind-Body Connection**: Chair yoga encourages you to connect to your body, mind, and breath. By tuning into your bodily sensations, acknowledging your emotions, and focusing on your breath, you could cultivate a deeper thoughts-body connection. This connection can foster a more sense of self-consciousness, self-compassion, and emotional nice-being.

4. **Increased Energy and Vitality**: Chair yoga carries gentle movements and stretches that can help stimulate move, improve flexibility, and growth power degrees. By undertaking those practices, you may experience a revitalizing effect on each of your body and mind, leading to advanced emotional nice-being.

5. **Relaxation and Mindfulness**: Chair yoga regularly includes relaxation and mindfulness sports, such as guided imagery and meditation. These practices can help calm the mind, reduce anxiety, and promote an experience of relaxation and inner peace. By incorporating these strategies into your chair yoga practice, you could beautify your emotional well-being.

Remember, chair yoga is not pretty much bodily fitness however also approximately nurturing your emotional nicely-being. So, embrace the practice, concentrate on your frame, and allow yourself to experience the transformative benefits it is able to offer.

Keep working towards chair yoga and nurturing your emotional well-being! □

Chair Yoga for Stress Relief

⬜Chair yoga is a remarkable practice for strain comfort. Here's why it can help you unwind and find a few an awful lot-wished calm:

1. **Gentle Movements:** Chair yoga includes gentle and reachable movements which might be suitable for all health degrees. These actions assist launch anxiety on your muscle groups, selling relaxation and decreasing physical stress.

2. **Deep Breathing**: Chair yoga emphasizes deep, mindful respiration techniques. By focusing on your breath and taste in gradual, intentional inhales and exhales, you activate your frame's rest response, which can assist alleviate pressure and anxiety.

3. **Mindfulness and Presence**: Engaging in chair yoga encourages you to be fully gifted within the second. By directing your interest to the sensations to your frame as you flow through the poses, you can let go of worries and distractions, fostering a sense of calm and peace.

4. **Stress Reduction Techniques**: Chair yoga consists of numerous strain reduction strategies, inclusive of guided

imagery and innovative muscle rest. These strategies permit you to launch tension, quiet your thoughts, and promote a state of deep relaxation.

5. **Overall Well-being**: Chair yoga is not just about bodily motion; it is a holistic exercise that addresses your ordinary nicely-being. By taking time for yourself, undertaking self-care, and prioritizing your intellectual and emotional fitness, you may effectively manipulate pressure and sell an experience of balance and concord in your lifestyles.

So, in case you're looking for a way to alleviate pressure, chair yoga is a brilliant preference. Give it a strive, and allow yourself to revel in the soothing effects it could have for your thoughts, frame, and soul. Remember, it is all approximately locating that inner peace and taking care of yourself. □

Chapter 8:
Chair Yoga for a Lifetime

Chair yoga is a fantastic practice that may be enjoyed all through a life-time. It offers severa benefits for human beings of every age, consisting of seniors. Here's why chair yoga is best for retaining health and properly-being as you journey via lifestyles:

1. **Accessibility**: Chair yoga is an incredibly handy shape of workout. It gets rid of the need to get down at the ground, making it appropriate for individuals with mobility limitations or stability issues. The use of a chair provides balance and guide, allowing you to quite simply have interaction in the exercise.

2. **Gentle and Low-Impact**: Chair yoga focuses on mild moves and poses that are clean at the joints. It allows you to improve flexibility, energy, and balance without setting stress for your body. This makes it an excellent desire for seniors or absolutely everyone seeking out a mild workout choice.

3. **Mind-Body Connection**: Chair yoga emphasizes the mind-body connection, promoting mindfulness and self-recognition. By practicing mindful respiration and being found in each

motion, you could domesticate a deeper experience of relaxation and internal peace.

4. **Improved Flexibility and Range of Motion**: Regular exercise of chair yoga can beautify flexibility and grow your variety of movement. The gentle stretches and moves assist to loosen tight muscles and enhance joint mobility, promoting universal physical well-being.

5. **Stress Relief and Relaxation**: Chair yoga contains relaxation strategies, along with deep respiratory and meditation, that may assist reduce strain and sell relaxation. Taking time for yourself and engaging in this practice can have an effective effect on your mental and emotional well-being.

Remember, chair yoga is a flexible practice that adapts for your needs and competencies. It's a lifelong journey that allows you to live active, maintain flexibility, and nurture your average properly-being. So, clutch a chair and embark on this pleasurable and enriching exercise at any stage of life! □

Incorporating Chair Yoga into Daily Life

☐Incorporating chair yoga into your each day existence is a awesome way to acquire its blessings. Here are some easy recommendations to help you make chair yoga a ordinary part of your recurring:

1. **Schedule Regular Practice**: Set aside specific times in your day for chair yoga. It could be in the morning to energize yourself or inside the night to unwind. Consistency is key, so goal for at least a few minutes of exercise every day.

2. **Start with a Warm-Up**: Begin your chair yoga session with gentle heat-up sporting activities. This could involve neck and shoulder rolls, wrist and ankle circles, or even seated marching. These moves help put together your body for the exercise ahead.

3. **Focus on Seated Postures**: Explore one of a kind seated postures for the duration of your chair yoga exercise. This can encompass sitting upright with proper alignment, crossing your legs, or maybe sitting on the brink of the chair for a deeper stretch. Find what feels cushty and supportive for you.

4. **Incorporate Breathing Exercises**: Integrate deep respiration physical games into your chair yoga routine. Take slow, deep

breaths, filling your stomach with air and exhaling completely. This facilitates calm the mind, lessens stress, and enhances rest.

5. **Gentle Stretches and Strength-Building**: Engage in seated stretches that concentrate on exclusive regions of your body, which include the neck, shoulders, lower back, and legs. Additionally, include energy-building sports like seated leg lifts or arm curls, the use of mild weights or resistance bands.

6. **Enhance Balance and Coordination**: Practice seated stability physical activities to improve balance and coordination. This can involve lifting one foot off the ground whilst maintaining stability at the chair or practicing gentle seated twists to interact your middle.

7. **End with Relaxation and Meditation**: Dedicate the last few minutes of your chair yoga practice to rest and meditation. Close your eyes, recognize your breath, and permit yourself to unwind. You also can comprise guided meditation or visualization techniques to decorate rest.

Remember, the splendor of chair yoga lies in its adaptability. Feel free to alter poses and movements to suit your comfort level and physical abilities.

Enjoy the journey of incorporating chair yoga into your everyday life, and permit it to convey a sense of peace, stability, and nice-being. □

Staying Motivated and Consistent

☐Staying encouraged and steady is prime in relation to any exercise, inclusive of chair yoga. Here are a few guidelines that will help you stay on target:

1. **Set Clear Goals**: Define what you want to reap through your chair yoga exercise. Whether it's enhancing flexibility, decreasing stress, or increasing energy, having clear goals will preserve your influence and provide you with something to work toward.

2. **Create a Routine**: Establish an everyday agenda in your chair yoga exercise. Consistency is essential, so discover a time that works quality for you and keep on with it. It could be in the morning, throughout a damage, or within the nighttime. Make it a non-negotiable part of your day.

3. **Find Accountability**: Share your chair yoga journey with a pal or be a part of a network of like-minded people. Having a person to hold you accountable and proportion your progress with can provide motivation and assist.

4. **Mix it Up**: Keep your chair yoga exercise fresh and thrilling by means of attempting distinctive exercises, poses, or styles. You can discover new films or attend digital lessons to keep things exciting. Variety can prevent boredom and help you stay engaged.

5. **Track Your Progress**: Keep a magazine or use a tracking app to record your chair yoga periods and observe any improvements or milestones you attain. Seeing your progress through the years may be quite motivating and inspire you to keep going.

6. **Celebrate Small Wins:** Acknowledge and celebrate your achievements alongside the way. Whether it's protecting a pose for a little longer or feeling greater comfortable, deliver yourself a pat at the return. Celebrating small wins boosts motivation and reinforces your commitment.

7. **Be Kind to Yourself:** Remember, it is everyday to have days whilst you senseless inspired or while lifestyles receives inside the way. Be gentle with yourself and do not beat yourself up over overlooked sessions. Just get back on target whilst you can and preserve shifting ahead.

By implementing those techniques, you may be able to live prompted and steady to your chair yoga practice. Embrace the adventure, revel in the benefits, and maintain up the terrific work! □

Resources for Further Exploration

If you are seeking to dive deeper into chair yoga and expand your knowledge, there are masses of sources available for similarly exploration. Here are some tips:

1. **Books**: Check out "Chair Yoga: Sit, Stretch, and Strengthen Your Way to a Happier, Healthier You" through Kristin McGee or "Gentle Yoga for Seniors" by way of Lanita Varshell. These books offer exact commands, illustrations, and adjustments especially tailored for seniors practicing chair yoga.

2. **Online Videos**: YouTube is a treasure trove of chair yoga movies. Look for channels like Yoga With Adriene, SilverSneakers, or the legit Yoga for Seniors channel. These movies provide guided chair yoga classes that you can comply with together with from the comfort of your property.

3. **Virtual Classes:** Many yoga studios and health facilities now offer virtual training, such as chair yoga. Check with neighborhood studios in your location or seek online platforms like Zoom or Mindbody for digital chair yoga instructions. These stay periods provide the possibility to have interaction with instructors and fellow individuals.

4. **Senior Centers or Community Centers:** Reach out to senior facilities or network centers on your neighborhood region. They frequently offer chair yoga training in particular designed for seniors. These in-individual instructions offer a supportive and social environment to exercise chair yoga.

5. **Mobile Apps:** Explore mobile apps that offer kind of yoga practices, together with chair yoga, with customizable capabilities consisting of duration, problem stage, and precise cognizance regions.

Don't forget, it's usually a terrific concept to discuss with a healthcare professional before starting any new exercise program, specifically if you have any pre-existing clinical conditions. Enjoy your exploration of chair yoga and feature a laugh discovering new resources! □

Conclusion

Congratulations! You've reached the end of this book on chair yoga for seniors over 60. Throughout these pages, we've got explored the notable types of chair yoga, specializing in seated postures, respiratory sports, mild stretches, energy-constructing sports, balance and coordination, and relaxation and meditation.

I desire this book has supplied you with valuable insights and realistic steerage on how to include chair yoga into your daily routine. Remember, chair yoga is a mild and reachable form of workout which can help enhance flexibility, power, and basic well-being.

But our journey doesn't end here. If you are hungry for extra information and need to preserve your exploration of chair yoga, I encourage you to always come lower back to check out my new releases.

Also Books, online videos, digital training, senior facilities, and mobile apps can all be fantastic avenues for similarly mastering and practice.

Always recall to concentrate on your frame, alter poses as needed, and visit a healthcare expert when you have any concerns or medical situations. Chair yoga is a stunning manner to honor and care for your frame, mind, and spirit.

Thank you for becoming a member of me on this chair yoga adventure. I hope you find joy, peace, and rejuvenation through your endured exercise. Wishing you many completely happy moments of chair yoga!"

NOTES

www.ingramcontent.com/pod-product-compliance
Lightning Source LLC
Chambersburg PA
CBHW081808250726
48653CB00010B/3842